Total Health Transformation : Fast guide to smart meal plan

Sharon S. Lent

Scan me

Gain more access to healthier books

TABLE OF CONTENTS

Green smoothie

White smoothie

Red smoothie

CHAPTER 6:Breakfast ideals

Bullet coffee

Keto coconut porridge

Keto Granola

Avocado Coconut smoothie

Crustless Quiche

Scrambled Bacon and egg

Flaxseed porridge

Veggies omelet

Greek yogurt parfait

CHAPTER 7: Lunch ideal

Broccoli bites

90 second bread turkey burgers

Chicken and Avocado boats

Beef sizzle and fathead pizza

Pesto chicken bakes

Cheesesteak Roll up

CHAPTER 8: Dinner ideals

Keto bread

Keto fish and chips

Thai red curry beef with broccoli rice

Salmon in Garlic butter with roasted asparagus

Peanut butter chicken curry

Keto pizza

Skirt steak and mushroom sauce

CONCLUSION

ABOUT THE AUTHOR

REVIEW

INTRODUCTION

In the bustling corridors of the medical world, where scrubs and stethoscopes ruled, there lived a resilient soul named Sharon S. Lent. She wasn't just a medical professional; she was a warrior on a personal battlefield—battling her own struggles with food and body image.

As Sharon walked those sterile halls, her journey was like an untold story, a narrative of silent battles fought within. In a world where scrutiny seemed to overshadow compassion, her fellow medical comrades cast judgments on her food choices and body structure. The whispers of criticism stung, echoing in the chambers of white-coated camaraderie.

But Sharon was no stranger to adversity. Instead of succumbing to the weight of judgment, she decided to pen a different chapter for herself. One day, fueled by a spark of determination, she embarked on a journey of self-discovery, making a conscious choice about the fuel her body would receive.

The narrative shifted as Sharon became the heroine of her own story. She explored the realms of mindful nourishment, transforming her relationship with food. The skeptics turned silent witnesses to a remarkable evolution. Sharon's journey, once marked by mockery, blossomed into a saga of triumph and resilience.

And so, "Total Health Transformation" was born—not just a book but a testament to Sharon's unwavering spirit. Within its pages, she shares the highs and lows, the victories and defeats, turning her struggles into a guide for those seeking their own transformation.

Join Sharon in this compelling tale of redemption, where the battle against judgment and self-doubt becomes a triumphant narrative of empowerment and wellness. "Total Health Transformation" is more than a book; it's the story of a warrior who decided to rewrite her script and emerged not just victorious but an inspiration for others daring to embark on their own transformative journey.

CHAPTER: 1 STORY ON THE WHOLE BODY RESET DIET

In the whole body reset Sharon S. Lent unfolds a captivating narrative of her personal odyssey toward total health transformation. Sharon, once ensnared by the complexities of modern life and a sedentary routine, discovered the transformative power of a holistic approach to wellness.

The story begins with Sharon's realization that the key to vitality lies in understanding the intricate interplay between nutrition, physical activity. She invites readers into her own journey the struggles, the aha moments, and the triumphs that ultimately led to her "TOTAL HEALTH TRANSFORMATION".

As the protagonist of her own story, Sharon doesn't just share her success; she extends a guiding hand to the reader. With meticulous detail, she unveils the Whole Body Reset Diet a roadmap to revitalization that goes beyond mere weight loss. Through a series of carefully crafted chapters Sharon takes readers on a step-by-step expedition, demystifying the principles of mindful nutrition, introducing an invigorating exercise routine.

Sharon understands that each reader is on a unique quest, and her approach is one of inclusivity. The diet is not a rigid set of rules but a flexible framework tailored to individual needs. The pages are adorned with mouthwatering recipes, accessible workout routines, and mindfulness exercises each designed to empower the reader to become the architect of their health transformation.

The journey doesn't merely focus on external changes; it delves into the profound connection between mind and body. As the narrative unfolds, readers find themselves not just following a diet but immersing in a lifestyle a paradigm shift towards lasting health and well-being.

As the story concludes, the reader is left inspired, equipped, and ready to embark on their personal journey to total health transformation. Sharon S. Lent becomes not just an author but a guiding companion, offering a narrative that transcends the pages, resonating in the daily choices and newfound vitality of those who embark on their Whole Body Reset journey.

What Is The
Whole Body Reset Diet

The whole Body Reset Diet is like an infinite Ctrl+Alt+Delete for your body, an amicable ensemble coordinated ordinarily culinary wizards. Envision it as a fantastic house cleaning occasion, where everywhere of your being gets a celebrity makeover. This isn't your all around average eating regimen; it's an all encompassing revival, a reset button for the whole ensemble of organs that make up the human body.

Picture your body as a clamoring city, every organ assuming an essential part in the day to day buzzing about. The Whole Body Reset Diet, on the other hand, does not intend to impose a dictatorial regime on this bustling city. All things being equal, it's even more an insightful metropolitan recharging project - rejuvenating neighborhoods, updating framework, and advancing a better, more energetic local area inside.

At its center, this diet is a festival of equilibrium. It's about creating a menu that flows like a well-choreographed dance, with flavors and macronutrients dancing gracefully alongside micronutrients. Not any more conflicting notes of overindulgence or the quiet murmur of supplement inadequacies - it's a culinary concerto where every fixing adds to the general show-stopper.

Presently, we should discuss the headliners in this excellent ensemble - the recipes. These are not simply culinary manifestations; they're masterpieces created with the accuracy of a stone carver and the energy of a maestro. From the lively servings of mixed greens that burst forward like a kaleidoscope to the good stews that warm the spirit, every recipe is a part in the legendary story of your body's restoration.

However, don't be tricked into thinking this is an excursion of hardship. God help us, the Entire Body Reset Diet is more similar to a well disposed guide driving you through a clamoring food market. It invites you to savor the diverse flavors and textures that nature has to offer and encourages you to explore the richness of whole, unprocessed foods. An update sustaining your body can be a great experience, not an errand.

Humane eating is what sets this diet apart. There's really no need to focus on unbending guidelines and culpability instigating limitations; it's tied in with producing an empathetic relationship with the food you devour. Like having a shrewd culinary coach urges you to stand by listening to your body's signs, directing you to settle on decisions that resound with your prosperity.

Humor is the mysterious fixing sprinkled liberally all through the Entire Body Reset Diet. It's the joy of savoring a dish that is perfectly imperfect, the laughs shared over a mishap with a new ingredient, and the laughter that bubbles up as you experiment in the kitchen. This diet recognizes that life is intended to be delighted in, as is the food on your plate.

The Entire Body Reset Diet is a groundbreaking excursion, for your constitution as well as for your relationship with food. It's tied in with squeezing the reset button, not out of distress, but rather out of adoration for the extraordinary machine that is your body. It's a merciful hug of wellbeing, health, and the sheer delight of enjoying each flavorful snapshot of this culinary experience called life.

EXERCISE AND SLEEP

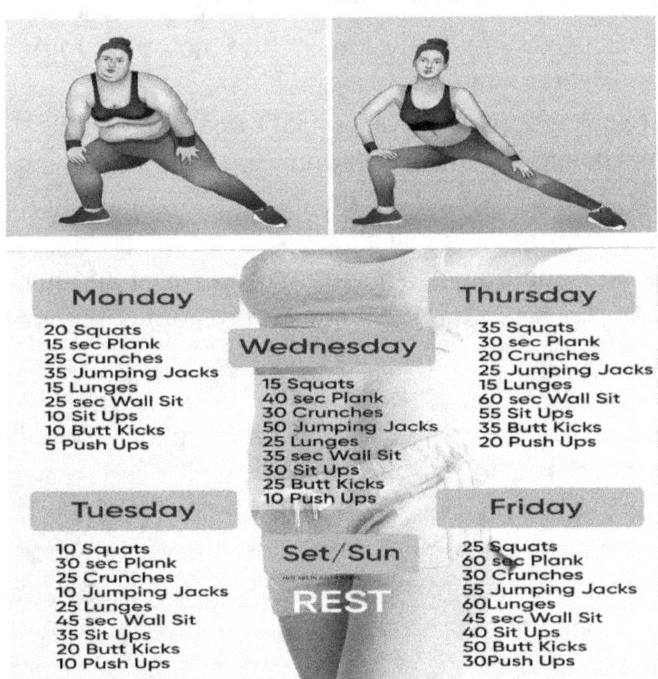

Embarking on the journey of weight loss and sculpting that coveted flat belly is a dynamic expedition, where exercise and sleep play pivotal roles as your trusty companions.

Imagine exercise as the sculptor and sleep as the rejuvenating artist—both working in tandem to carve out the masterpiece that is a healthier, fitter you. When you hit the gym or engage in physical activity, it's not merely about burning calories; it's a symphony of movements that revitalize your body, igniting the metabolic furnace.

Exercise becomes the alchemist transforming sweat into the elixir of strength, endurance, and a metabolism that hums like a well-tuned engine. From heart-thumping cardio to muscle-chiseling strength training, each session contributes to the grand narrative of shedding weight and revealing the sleek contours of a flat belly.

Lack of sleep, on the other hand, plays the villain, disrupting this delicate choreography. It's like throwing a wrench into the gears of a well-oiled machine, with consequences ranging from increased cravings for sugary snacks to a sluggish metabolism that hampers weight loss efforts.

Quality sleep isn't just a luxury; it's a strategic necessity in the battle for a flat belly. It's during these nocturnal hours that your body, like a diligent sculptor putting finishing touches, trims excess fat and fortifies your resolve to stick to a healthier lifestyle.

In essence, exercise and sleep are the dynamic duo, the Batman and Robin of your weight loss journey. While exercise reshapes and tones, sleep ensures the body's intricate machinery functions optimally, supporting your quest for that flat belly.

So, lace up those sneakers, hit the gym, relish the post-workout glow, and when night falls, surrender to the embrace of a good night's sleep. Together, they form the formidable alliance that will not only redefine your physique but also escort you to the promised land of a slimmer waistline and a flatter belly. It's not just a journey; it's a transformational odyssey, where exercise and sleep become your unwavering allies in the pursuit of a healthier, happier you.

CHAPTER: 2 BENEFITS OF THE WHOLE BODY RESET DIET

The Whole Body Reset Diet offers a complete way to deal with wellbeing, advancing various advantages. By stressing supplement thick food sources, it upholds weight the executives and upgrades energy levels. This diet focuses on entire, natural food sources, encouraging better processing and stomach wellbeing. With an emphasis on hydration, it supports detoxification, advancing more clear skin and further developed organ capability The whole Body Reset Diet can emphatically influence mental prosperity, lessening irritation and supporting mental capability. By empowering a reasonable and practical way to deal with eating, this diet lays out solid propensities, cultivating long haul health and strength.

Assist you in losing weight

The whole Body Reset Diet fills in as a strong partner in weight reduction by tending to different features of wellbeing. Above all else, it accentuates supplement thick, entire food varieties, which advance satiety and diminish generally caloric admission. This not only helps you lose weight, but it also makes sure that the body gets the vitamins and minerals it needs to work well.

It is essential to emphasize hydration. Sufficient water consumption upholds digestion, helping the body effectively consume calories. The diet's emphasis on cutting out processed foods and sugars helps keep blood sugar levels in check and prevents insulin spikes that can cause fat storage.

By focusing on lean proteins and fiber-rich food sources, the whole Body Reset Diet upholds muscle upkeep and advances a sensation of totality. This deters gorging and keeps a calorie shortfall essential for shedding overabundance weight.

The regard for stomach wellbeing is another key element. A reasonable stomach microbiome is related with a better digestion, and by consolidating probiotic-rich food sources, the eating regimen supports keeping up with this equilibrium.

The whole Body Reset Diet offers an all encompassing way to deal with weight reduction, tending to dietary decisions, hydration, and stomach wellbeing to make a supportable and viable technique for shedding pounds and advancing generally speaking prosperity.

Provide highly nutritious food

The Whole Body Reset Diet is like having a team of nutritional superheroes over to eat dinner with you—each dish packs a powerful punch of health benefits. Picture it as a culinary transformation, where each feast is an essential collusion of flavors and supplements intended to fuel your body's true capacity.

In this gastronomic excursion, products of the soil become your brilliant partners, flooding your plate with nutrients and cell reinforcements that safeguard your body from the everyday routine. Fit proteins step in as the muscle-manufacturers, guaranteeing your solidarity and essentialness.

Entire grains, the uncelebrated yet truly great individuals of this nourishing adventure, bring supported energy and fiber, supporting your stomach related framework and keeping those food cravings under control. Solid fats, the savvy tutors in this dietary experience, guide you toward a reasonable methodology, feeding your cerebrum and heart.

You're not just eating as you enjoy the pleasures of this full-body feast; you're furnishing your body with an orchestra of supplements. It's anything but an eating regimen; it's a wholesome romantic tale, where each nibble is a token of care, reviving your general existence. The Entire Body Reset Diet isn't just about what you eat; it's a festival of giving your body the healthy sustenance it desires, making ready for a renewed and strong you.

CHAPTER: 3
FUNDAMENTAL OF THE WHOLE BODY RESET

The fundamental principles of the Whole Body Reset are designed to improve overall health and well-being. At its center, this approach stresses entire, natural food varieties, controlling people from refined sugars and exceptionally handled choices. The emphasis is on devouring supplement thick food varieties, including various natural products, vegetables, lean proteins, and entire grains.

Hydration assumes a critical part in the major standards of the Entire Body Reset. Sufficient water admission upholds processing, supplement ingestion, and poison end. This emphasis on hydration helps the body function and feel alive overall.

The eating regimen energizes careful eating and part control, encouraging a fair and maintainable relationship with food. By focusing on higher standards without ever compromising, people can accomplish satiety through supplement rich choices, advancing a better body creation.

The Entire Body Reset likewise coordinates the significance of stomach wellbeing. Probiotic-rich food varieties are incorporated to help a fair microbiome, emphatically influencing processing and generally invulnerable capability.

The basic standards of the Entire Body Reset line up with a comprehensive and practical way to deal with sustenance, expecting to feed the body with fundamental supplements, advance hydration, and lay out careful dietary patterns for long haul prosperity.

How to follow the whole body reset diet

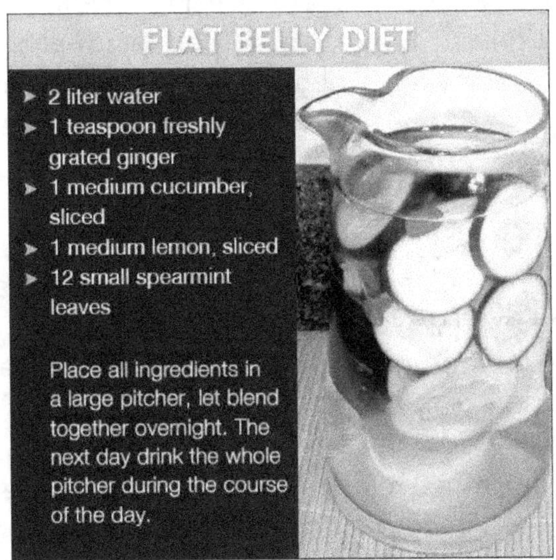

To Successfully follow the whole Body Reset Diet, start by focusing on entire, natural food varieties. Include healthy fats, lean proteins, whole grains, and a variety of colorful fruits and vegetables in your meals. Limit or kill handled food varieties, refined sugars, and counterfeit added substances. Embrace cooking at home to have more noteworthy command over fixings and part estimates.

Hydration is vital; mean to drink a lot of water over the course of the day. This supports assimilation, supplement ingestion, and detoxification - necessary parts of the Entire Body Reset.

Practice careful eating by focusing on yearning and totality signals. Stay away from interruptions while eating and enjoy each nibble. Select more modest, more continuous feasts to keep up with consistent energy levels.

Integrate probiotic-rich food varieties like yogurt, kefir, and matured vegetables to advance a solid stomach microbiome. To support muscle maintenance and satiety, give lean proteins like poultry, fish, beans, and legumes priority.

Explore different avenues regarding assorted recipes to keep dinners intriguing and keep up with adherence to the arrangement. Standard active work supplements the Entire Body Reset, adding to by and large wellbeing and weight the executives.

Keep in mind, consistency is vital. Make gradual adherence to these tenets and lifestyle adjustments that are long-lasting for long-term success. Talking with a medical services proficient or nutritionist can give customized direction, guaranteeing the Entire Body Reset lines up with your singular necessities and objectives.

CHAPTER: 4
What food to eat

How Much Water to Drink a Day?

Body Weight lbs	Fluid # ounces	# 8 ounce Glasses of water
50 lb	25-50 oz	3-6
75 lb	38-75 oz	5-9
100 lb	50-100 oz	6-13
125 lb	63-125 oz	8-16
150 lb	75-150 oz	9-19
175 lb	88-175 oz	11-22
200 lb	100-200 oz	13-25
225 lb	113-225 oz	14-28
250 lb	125-250 oz	16-31
275 lb	138-275 oz	17-34
300 lb	150-300 oz	19-38
325 lb	163-325 oz	20-41
350 lb	175-350 oz	22-44

agelessinvesting.com

On this journey to weight loss and a flat stomach, I am your reliable guide. Priorities straight, we should discuss your plate. Top it off with vivid veggies like mixed greens, ringer peppers, and broccoli. These supplement pressed ponders support your digestion as well as keep you full longer.

Let's talk about lean proteins now. Tofu, turkey, fish, and chicken are your friends. They're like the superheroes of your eating regimen, assisting you with building muscle and consume fat. What's more, remember the eggs - they're a force to be reckoned with of supplements.

Your dependable allies are whole grains. Decide on quinoa, earthy colored rice, and oats. They give enduring energy, keeping those food cravings under control. Ditch the refined carbs - they're the lowlifes attacking your level midsection mission.

Solid fats, similar to avocados, nuts, and olive oil, are your clear-cut advantage. They keep your skin sparkling and your digestion murmuring. Simply hold segments within proper limits - even superheroes need to watch their admission.

Hydration is your companion in wrongdoing battling. Water is essential for flushing toxins and maintaining a healthy metabolism. Avoid sugary beverages; they're like kryptonite for your objectives.

Fruits, Greek yogurt, or a handful of nuts are smart snacks. They fulfill desires without crashing your excursion. Also, with regards to sweet treats, dim chocolate is your irreproachable extravagance.

Keep in mind, consistency is your most prominent partner. Practice these decisions all the time, and you'll shake that level stomach superhuman style. Cheers to your wellbeing process!

What food to avoid

Beware of sugary drinks; they're like cunning adversaries trying to undermine your progress. Opt for water or herbal teas instead to stay hydrated without the added calories.

Steer clear of refined carbs – the refined sugar, white bread, and pastries are like the villains plotting against your flat belly aspirations. Choose whole grains for a healthier alternative.

Watch out for excessive sodium in processed snacks and canned goods; they're like silent saboteurs causing bloating and water retention. Opt for fresh, whole foods to avoid this trap.

Say no to trans fats found in many fried and packaged foods – they're the masked villains harming your heart health and sabotaging your weight loss efforts. Choose healthier cooking methods and natural fats instead.

Processed meats are like tricky adversaries disguising themselves as protein sources. Opt for lean proteins like chicken, turkey, or plant-based alternatives to stay on track.

Avoid late-night snacking; it's the shadowy enemy that can disrupt your sleep and hinder your progress. Opt for a cup of herbal tea or a small, healthy snack if hunger strikes.

Remember, knowledge is your superpower. Arm yourself with awareness, and you'll navigate through the temptations on your journey to a healthier, flatter you. Stay resilient!

CHAPTER: 5 Smoothie
Green smoothie

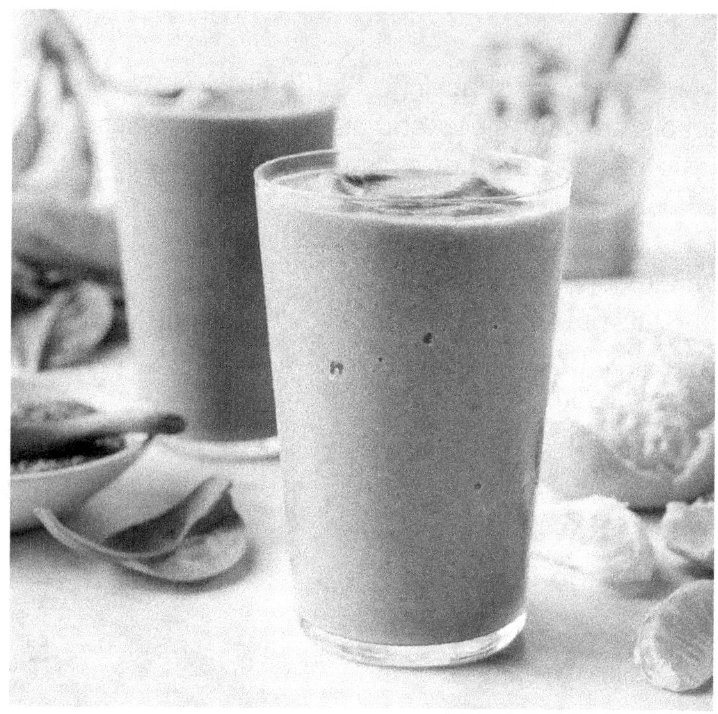

INGREDIENTS

2 cups spinach
2 cups water
1 cup mango
1 cup pineapple

2 bananas (Use at least one frozen fruit to chill your smoothie. We often use frozen mangos and bananas our green smoothies.)

INSTRUCTIONS
Tightly pack 2 cups of leafy greens in a measuring cup and then toss into a blender.

Add water and blend together until all leafy chunks are gone.

Add mango, pineapple and bananas and blend again until smooth.

Pour into a mason jar (or cute cup of your choice).
Gulp or sip like a rawkstar!

Health Benefit

Nutrient Powerhouse: Green smoothies are loaded with vitamins, minerals, and antioxidants from leafy greens and fruits. These nutrients support your overall health and metabolism.

Fiber Boost: The fiber content in green smoothies is a game-changer. Fiber keeps you full, curbing unnecessary snacking and promoting a feeling of satiety, crucial for weight loss.

Hydration Helper: Many green smoothie recipes include water or other hydrating liquids. Proper hydration aids digestion and can prevent overeating.

Low in Calories: If you focus on using mainly vegetables and moderate amounts of fruits in your green smoothies, they can be a low-calorie, nutrient-dense option. This is key for weight loss.

Metabolism Kickstart: Certain ingredients in green smoothies, like green tea or spicy additions, may give a gentle boost to your metabolism, aiding in the calorie-burning process.

White smoothie

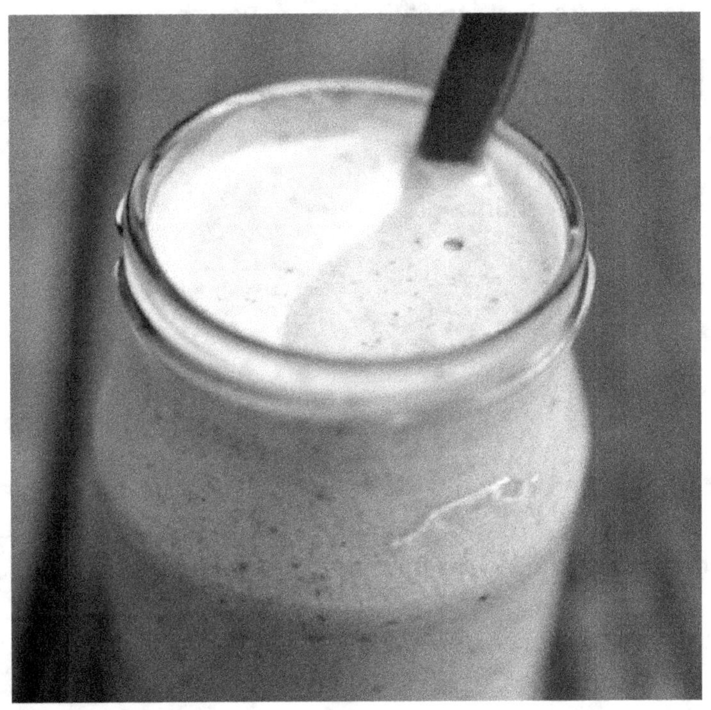

INGREDIENTS

3 tbsp. coconut puree best from Dr. Goerg

2 organic eggs raw

1 pear

1/2 - 1 banana

2 plums

if necessary some hemp seeds peeled, in raw food quality

approx. 150 ml water

INSTRUCTION

Cut the ingredients to fit the size of your blender.

Blend for 45-60 seconds until you reach a smooth, creamy consistency.

Enjoy with all your heart!

Health Benefit

Rich in Calcium: Dairy or yogurt in white smoothies contributes to a calcium boost, promoting strong bones and teeth. This is vital for overall skeletal health.

Protein Powerhouse: Yogurt, a common ingredient in white smoothies, is a great source of protein. Protein helps in muscle repair and growth, making it beneficial for those engaged in physical activities.

Gut-Friendly: Yogurt in white smoothies contains probiotics, fostering a healthy gut microbiome. A balanced gut contributes to improved digestion and better nutrient absorption.

Electrolyte Balance: Ingredients like coconut water or coconut milk add electrolytes to white smoothies, aiding in hydration and maintaining the body's fluid balance.

Heart Health Support: Unsaturated fats from ingredients like coconut can contribute to heart health by promoting healthy cholesterol levels.

Natural Sweetness: Bananas or other fruits often used in white smoothies provide natural sweetness without relying on added sugars. This makes them a sweet treat without the guilt.

Red Smoothie

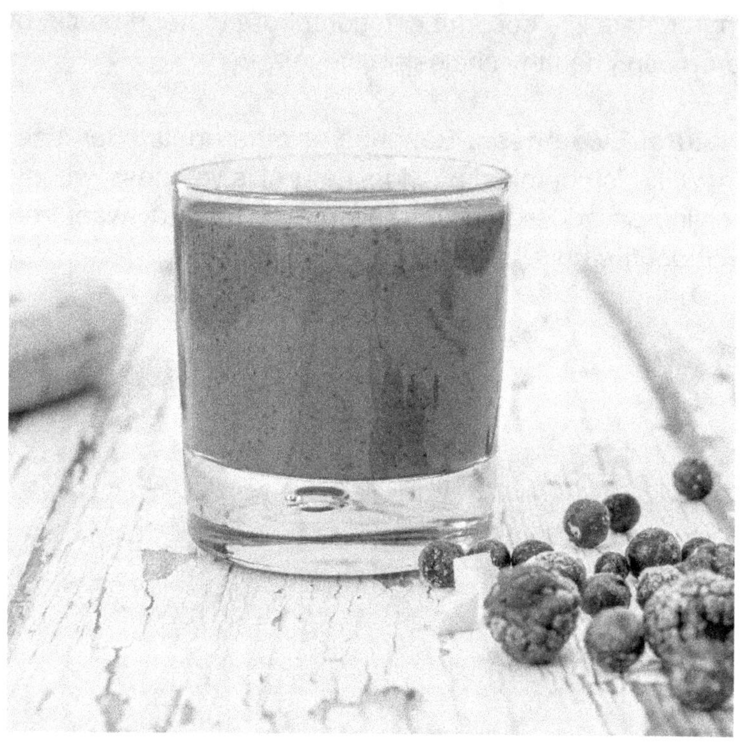

INGREDIENTS

1 (6 ounce) container fat-free strawberry yogurt
1 cup fat-free milk
1 ½ cups fresh sliced strawberries
½ cup fresh red raspberries
1 cup small ice cubes or crushed ice

INSTRUCTION

In a blender, combine yogurt, milk, and fruit. Cover and blend until smooth.

Add ice; cover and blend until almost smooth.

Health Benefits

Antioxidant Boost: Red berries such as strawberries, raspberries, and cranberries are rich in antioxidants. These compounds help combat oxidative stress, supporting overall health and potentially reducing the risk of chronic diseases.

Vitamin C Source: Berries, particularly strawberries, are high in vitamin C. This essential nutrient boosts the immune system, promotes skin health, and aids in collagen production.

Heart Health: The anthocyanins found in red berries may contribute to heart health by helping to lower blood pressure and reduce inflammation.

Fiber Content: Berries are an excellent source of dietary fiber. Fiber aids in digestion, promotes a feeling of fullness, and supports a healthy weight by regulating blood sugar levels.

Metabolism Boost: Some berries, like raspberries, contain compounds that may help boost metabolism. This can be beneficial for those aiming for weight management.

Blood Sugar Regulation: Berries have a low glycemic index, which means they have a minimal impact on blood sugar levels. This makes them a suitable choice for those managing diabetes or watching their sugar intake.

Low in Calories: Red berries, such as strawberries and raspberries, are naturally low in calories while being high in fiber. This makes them an excellent choice for those looking to manage their weight without compromising on taste.

Fiber for Satiety: Berries are rich in dietary fiber, which promotes a feeling of fullness. This can help control appetite, reducing the likelihood of overeating and supporting weight loss goals.

Nutrient Density: Red berries are packed with essential vitamins, minerals, and antioxidants. Despite being low in calories, they provide a concentrated dose of nutrients, supporting overall health during weight loss.

Hydration Support: Berries have a high water content, contributing to your daily hydration needs. Staying adequately hydrated is crucial for overall well-being and can support weight loss efforts.

Natural Sweetness: The natural sugars in red berries provide sweetness without the need for added sugars. This helps keep your overall sugar intake in check, promoting a healthier diet conducive to weight loss.

CHAPTER: 6 Breakfast ideals
Bullet coffee

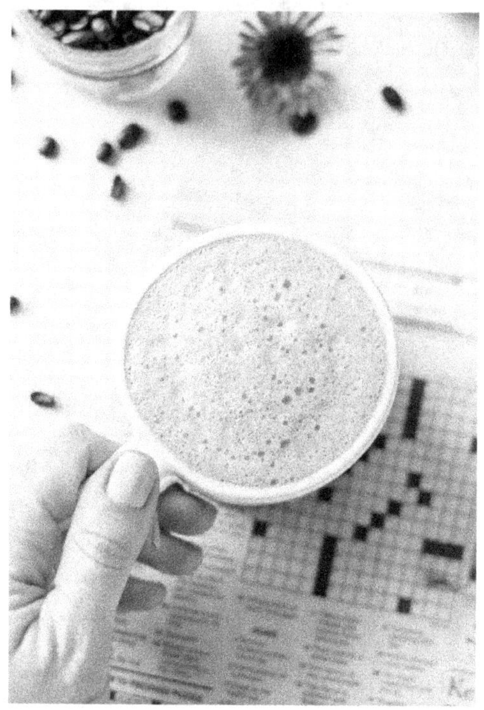

INGREDIENT

10–12 oz hot brewed coffee

1 tablespoon high quality fat of choice – butter, ghee, coconut oil, MCT oil, or cacao butter are all great choices

Pinch of sea salt (optional, but does bring the flavors together nicely and balance out some of the bitterness of the coffee)

Any adaptogens, herbs, supplements, flavors or sweeteners that you want to add (optional)

INSTRUCTIONS
Add all ingredients to a blender and blend on high until creamy and emulsified.
Pour into your favorite mug and enjoy!

NOTE
I usually use my blender, but if you don't have one (or don't feel like dirtying yours up), a great alternative is a battery operated milk frother. This milk frother from Amazon is less than $20 and it's the best one I've ever used.

Keto coconut porridge

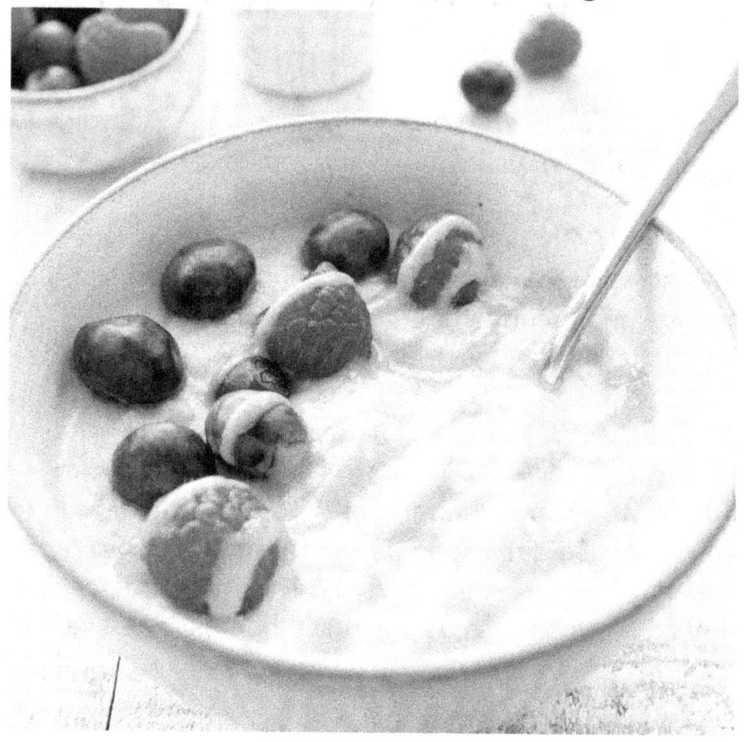

INGREDIENTS

1 egg, beaten
1 tbsp coconut flour
¼ tsp ground psyllium husk powder
¼ tsp salt
1 oz. butter or coconut oil
4 tbsp coconut cream

INSTRUCTIONS

In a small bowl, combine the egg, coconut flour, psyllium husk powder and salt.

Over low heat, melt the butter and coconut cream. Slowly whisk in the egg mixture, combining until you achieve a creamy, thick texture.

Serve with coconut milk or cream. Top your porridge with a few fresh or frozen berries and enjoy!

Keto Granola

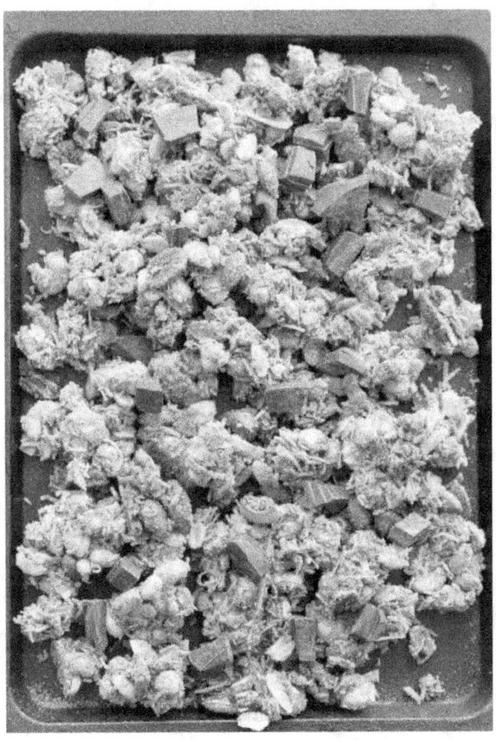

INGREDIENTS

1 1/2 cup nuts chopped roughly
1/2 cup almond flour
1 cup unsweetened shredded coconut
1/3 cup keto maple syrup can substitute for maple syrup
or agave nectar, if not keto.

INSTRUCTIONS

Preheat the oven to 180C/350F. Line a large baking tray
with parchment paper and set aside.

In a large mixing bowl, add all your dry ingredients and
mix well. Add your keto maple syrup and mix until fully
incorporated.

Transfer the granola mixture on the lined tray and
spread out in an even layer.

Bake for 15-20 minutes, stirring halfway through.
Granola is done when the edges have gone golden
brown.

Remove from the oven and allow to cool completely,
before breaking apart into desired size.

NOTE

TO STORE: Leftovers should always be kept in a
sealable container, at room temperature. Be sure there
is sealed properly, to avoid the keto granola softening.

TO FREEZE: This granola is freezer friendly and can be stored in the freezer. Place in a freezer friendly container and keep in the freezer for up to 6 months.

Avocado Coconut Smoothie

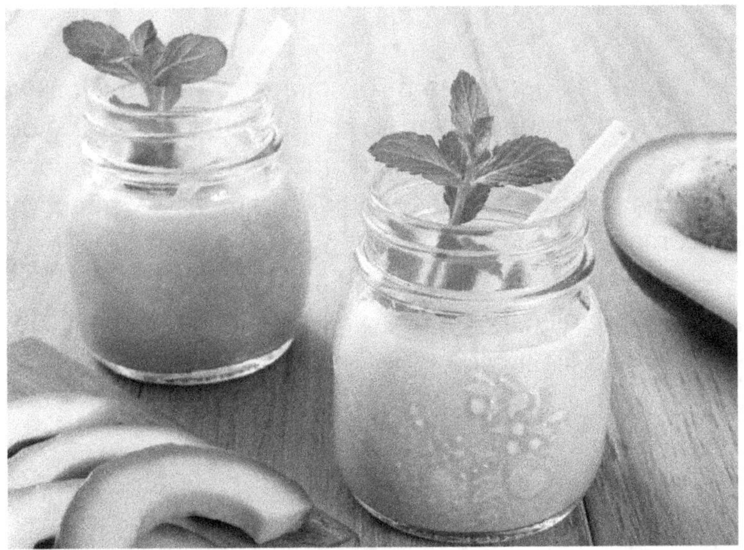

INGREDIENTS
8 ice cubes

1 medium avocado, diced

½ cup low-fat vanilla yogurt

½ cup whole milk

¼ cup cream of coconut

INSTRUCTIONS

Combine ice cubes, avocado, yogurt, milk, and cream of coconut in a blender; blend until smooth.

TIPS

Be sure to use cream of coconut. It's thick (like sweetened condensed milk) and may be found in your grocery store with the cocktail mixes. Don't use coconut milk or coconut water as that will dramatically affect the outcome.

Add more milk if you like your smoothie thinner. Add more ice if you like it thicker.

Crustless Quiche

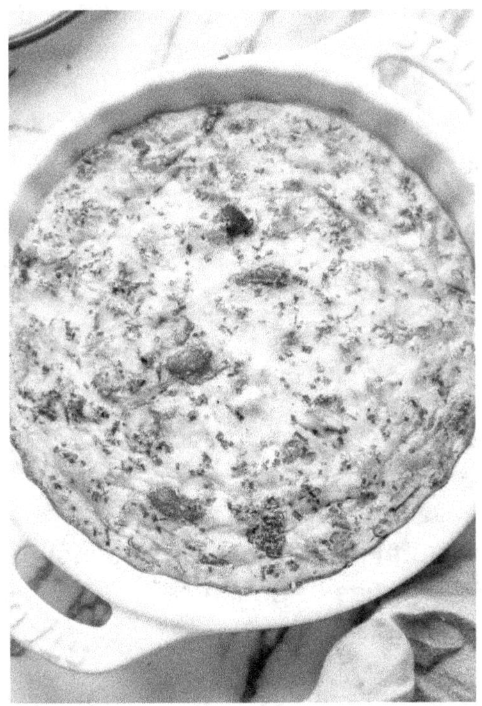

INGREDIENTS
FOR THE QUICHE BASE:
6 large eggs
2/3 cup whole milk
¼ cup half-and-half
½ teaspoon kosher salt
¼ teaspoon black pepper
1 teaspoon Dijon mustard optional
Pinch ground nutmeg optional

1 1/2 cups mix-ins of choice: See below for suggestions and ingredient notes for a broccoli bacon version if you are a little under or over 1 1/2 cups, that's OK
2/3 cup grated Gruyère cheese or swap fontina, sharp cheddar, or smoked mozzarella
2 tablespoons chopped fresh chives

FOR THE MIX-INS:
Cooked crumbled bacon
Chopped and sautéed broccoli
Caramelized onions
Cubed leftover ham
Roasted vegetables roughly chopped

INSTRUCTIONS
Place a rack in the center of your oven and preheat the oven to 350 degrees F. Coat a deep 9-inch pie dish with nonstick spray.

Prepare any mix-ins (see recipe notes for a broccoli bacon version and the blog post above for more suggestions).

In a large mixing bowl, whisk together the eggs, milk, half-and-half, salt, pepper, mustard, and nutmeg.
Scatter the mix-ins evenly across the bottom of the prepared pie dish.
Sprinkle the cheese on top.

Carefully pour the egg mixture into the dish. Place the dish on a rimmed baking sheet. Sprinkle the chives over the top.

Bake the quiche on the baking sheet until the center is set, about 35 minutes. It should look puffed and golden at the edges, and when a thin, sharp knife is inserted in the center, the center should be cooked through without visible liquid. Let cool a few minutes. Cut into big wedges. Enjoy warm.

NOTE

For the Broccoli Bacon version shown in this post: Chop 4 slices of thick-cut bacon into bite-sized pieces. Cook in a skillet over medium low heat, until the pieces are crisp and the fat has rendered, about 8 minutes. With a slotted spoon, remove the bacon to a towel-lined plate. Discard all but 1 tablespoon bacon fat from the skillet. Add 2 cups of small-chopped broccoli florets and 1 small, very thinly sliced red or yellow onion. Sauté until the onion is tender, about 10 minutes. Use in the quiche as directed.

TO STORE: Refrigerate quiche in an airtight storage container for up to 3 days.

TO REHEAT: Rewarm leftovers in a pie dish in the oven at 350 degrees F.

TO FREEZE: You can freeze a crustless quiche. Wrap the quiche tightly in plastic wrap and freeze in an airtight freezer-safe storage container for up to 3 months. Let thaw overnight in the refrigerator before reheating.

Scrambled Bacon and Eggs

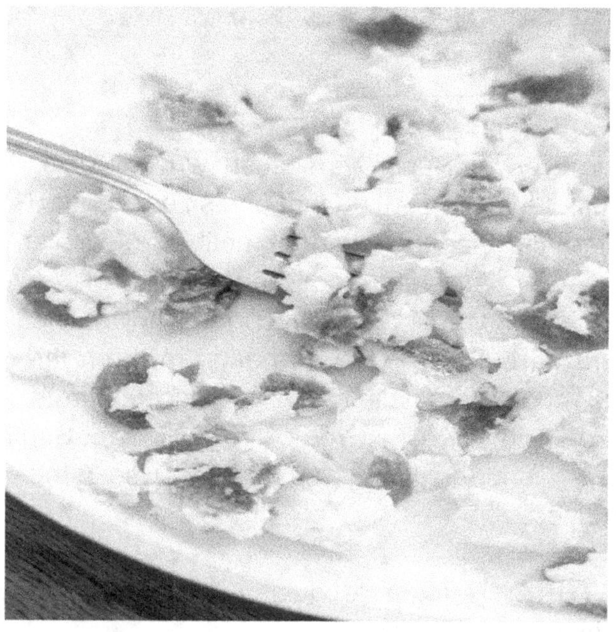

INGREDIENTS

3 pieces bacon pork or turkey
4 eggs
1 tablespoon milk
1/4 teaspoon salt

dash of pepper
1 tablespoon of butter

INSTRUCTIONS
Cook bacon according to directions on package. Once cooked cut the bacon up into 1/2 inch pieces.

Crack open eggs in small bowl. Add milk, salt, dash of pepper and bacon into bowl. Mix together until eggs are beaten.

Melt butter in skillet on medium high heat, making sure to coat the entire bottom of the pan. Add egg mixture to pan.

Once egg mixture seems to have set (about 4 minutes), break up with spatula to scramble and flip. Continue cooking and scrambling until eggs are fully cooked and no longer runny.

Serve and enjoy!

Flaxseed porridge

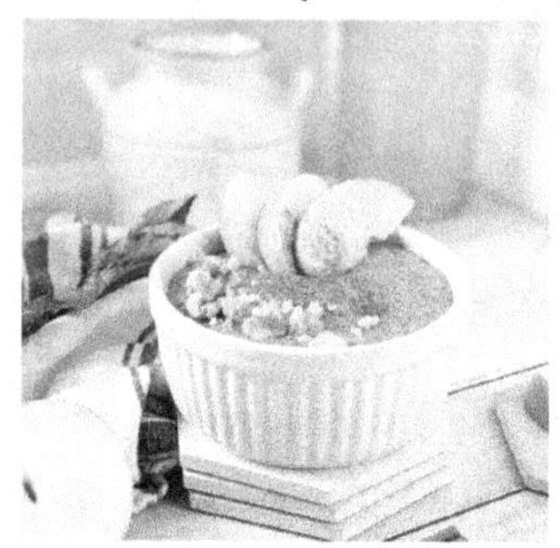

INGREDIENTS

1 cup plain unsweetened almond milk
1/4 cup flaxseeds
1/4 almond meal or crushed nuts (you can use any leftovers from making nut milk!)
1 tablespoon agave
1/2 teaspoon cinnamon
1/2 cup fruit I used sliced apples
Pinch salt
Nuts for garnish I used walnuts

INSTRUCTIONS

In a sauce pan, add all ingredients and heat on low. Constantly stir for a few minutes until the mixture is hot, but not quite bubbling.

Transfer warm porridge to a dish a garnish with extra fruit, cinnamon, and nuts if desired.

Enjoy!

Veggies Omelet

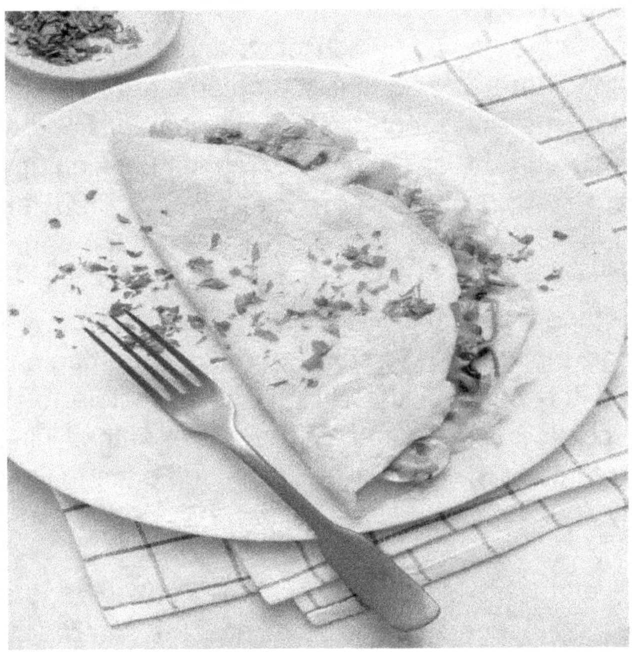

INGREDIENTS

1 tablespoon olive oil

¼ cup finely chopped red onions

¼ cup finely chopped red peppers

¼ cup sliced mushrooms

1 cup fresh baby spinach

salt and pepper to taste

2-3 eggs

1 tablespoon water

2 tablespoons shredded cheddar cheese

Fresh parsley for serving

INSTRUCTIONS

Heat olive oil in an 8-inch or 10-inch non-stick skillet over medium heat. Add the red onions, red peppers and mushrooms and cook until crisp tender, about 3-5 minutes. Add the spinach and continue cooking until the spinach wilts, about 1 more minute. Transfer the vegetables to a small bowl and wipe down the pan.

Crack and beat eggs with water in a small bowl. Pour the egg mixture in the same pan. As eggs begin to set around the edge of the skillet, use a spatula to gently push cooked portions toward the center of the skillet. Tilt and rotate the skillet to allow uncooked eggs to flow into empty spaces.

When eggs are almost set, add the cooked vegetables to half of the omelet and add the cheddar cheese on top. Place a spatula under the un-filled half, and fold over.

Gently slide from the skillet onto a plate. Season with salt and pepper and serve immediately top with fresh parsley

Greek yogurt parfait

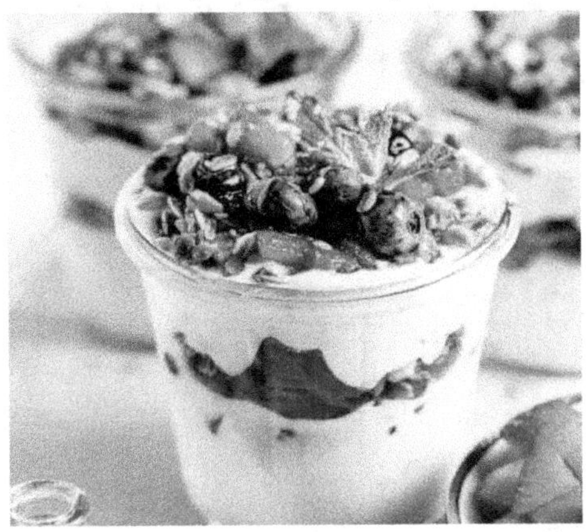

INGREDIENTS

1 tablespoon honey or maple syrup optional – more as a drizzle

¾ cup plain Greek yogurt

¼ cup berries or any other fruit cut into small 1-inch chunks

¼ cup homemade granola or store bought granola

INSTRUCTIONS

If using a sweetener, mix it with greek yogurt in a small bowl until fully combined.

To layer the yogurt parfait, place half of the yogurt at the bottom of a mason jar or a bowl. Top it off with half of the fruit and half of the granola. Cover them with the rest of the yogurt and top it off with the rest of the fruit and granola.

If preferred, finish it off with a drizzle of honey. Serve immediately.

CHAPTER : 7 Lunch ideals
Broccoli Bites

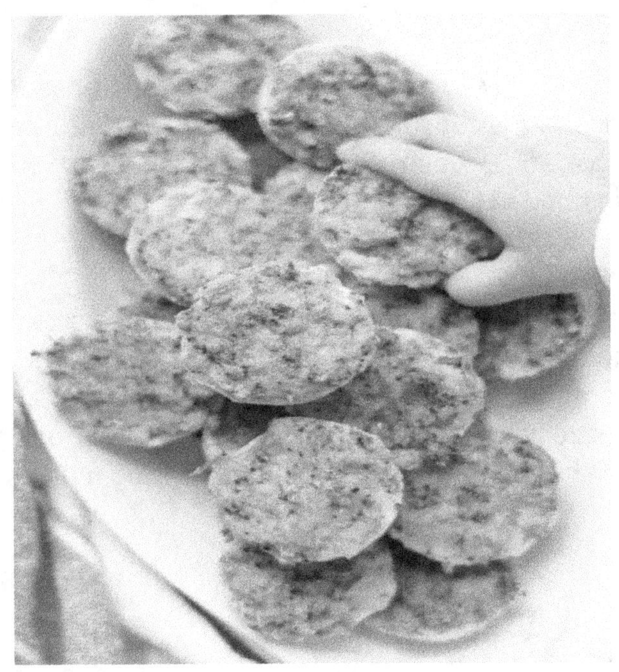

INGREDIENTS

Yes12 ounces frozen broccoli florets, thawed and patted dry

4 eggs, beaten

¼ cup whole wheat breadcrumbs

1 teaspoon garlic powder

1 teaspoon oregano

¾-1 cup shredded cheddar cheese

INSTRUCTIONS

Preheat oven to 375°F (190°C). Chop broccoli into small pieces. In a large mixing bowl, add the broccoli, eggs, breadcrumbs, cheese, and seasonings. Stir until well mixed.

Divide the broccoli mixture evenly into a greased, lined or silicone 12-cup muffin pan. Bake for 15-20 minutes until golden. Be sure to cook egg dishes to 160°F as recommended by the USDA.

NOTE
Transfer leftovers in an airtight container and store in the refrigerator for up to 5 days. Enjoy cold, at room temperature, or microwave briefly.
Or freeze for up to 2 months. I recommend using the flash freezing method that I use for freezing muffins.

90 Second bread turkey burgers

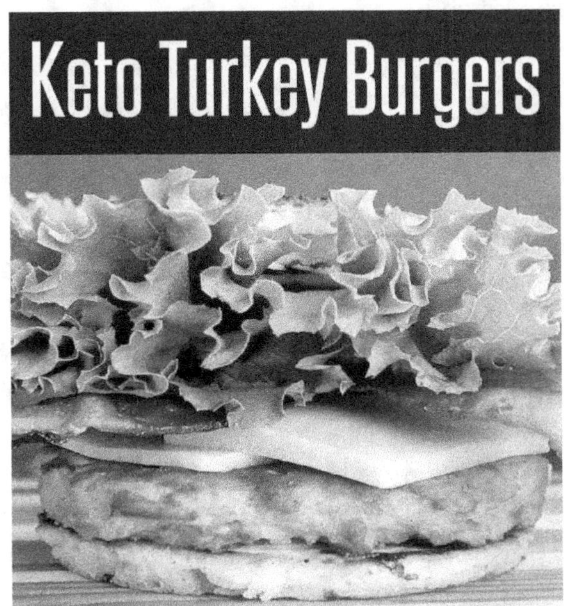

INGREDIENTS

Burgers

1-1.25 lbs ground turkey

1/4 cup diced onion

2 cloves minced garlic

1/2 cup low carb bbq sauce divided

1 egg

1/2 cup almond flour

1/4 tsp sea salt

1/4 tsp ground black pepper

4 90 Second Keto Breads

Optional Toppings

bacon

cheddar cheese
sugar free ketchup
mustard
pickles

EQUIPMENT NEEDED
Medium Bowl
Cutting Board and Knife
Baking Sheet with Non Stick Baking Mat
Meat Thermometer

INSTRUCTIONS
Heat oven to 375°. Dice up the onion and mince the garlic. In a medium bowl add the ground turkey, onion, garlic, egg, 1/4 cup Low Carb BBQ Sauce, 1/4 tsp sea salt, 1/4 tsp ground black pepper and almond flour.

Line a baking sheet with a non stick baking mat or parchment paper. Mix the burgers well then shape into four patties and place each evenly on the baking sheet. Bake for 10 minutes.

Brush the burgers well with the low carb bbq sauce, then bake for 5 minutes. Flip the burgers over, brush with more low carb bbq sauce and bake for 5-10 minutes until the internal temperature reaches 165°.

Five minutes before the burgers are fully cooked, make the 90 Second Keto Breads and prep the other choice ingredients.

When the Low Carb Turkey Burgers are fully cooked, build the burgers with your choice of spreads, sauces and other optional toppings! Yum!

Chicken and Avocado Boat

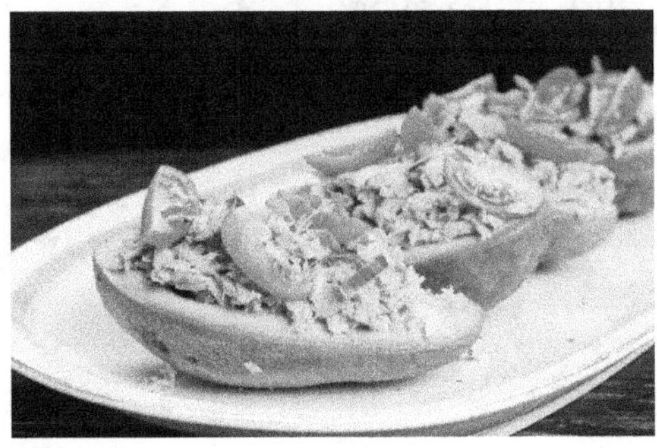

INGREDIENTS
2 avocados
2 grilled chicken breasts- cooked, shredded into small pieces
1/2 tsp basil
1/2 tsp thyme
3 tbsp cilantro
1/2 tsp garlic powder
2 Tbsp. lemon juice
1/2 tsp paprika
Salt and pepper to taste
1/4 cup red onion, diced
1 Tomato, small, diced
1 tsp olive oil.

INSTRUCTIONS

Cut avocados lengthwise and remove the pit. Scoop out the avocado to create a cavity. Lightly brush the avocado with olive oil to prevent browning. Mix shredded chicken, onions,tomatoes, all herbs, garlic powder and all other spices and lemon juice in a bowl. Adjust the lemon juice and spices to taste. Fill the chicken mixture in the avocado boat.

Serve it at your next party!

Beef sizzle fathead pizza

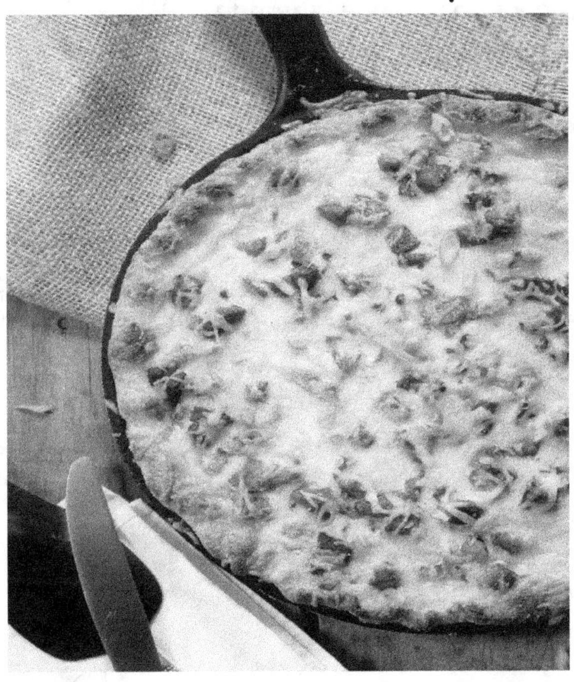

INGREDIENTS
FOR THE DOUGH:
2 oz cream cheese
2 cups mozzarella, shredded
2 eggs, beaten
1 cup almond flour
Salt and pepper, to taste
FOR THE TOPPINGS:
2 eggs
6 strips bacon, cooked
1/2 pound sausage, cooked

1/2 cup mozzarella cheese, shredded
1/4 cup cheddar cheese, shredded
2 green onions, chopped

INSTRUCTIONS
Preheat oven to 400, grease a cast iron pan.
For the dough:

Mix cream cheese and mozzarella together in a bowl. You can optionally microwave for 1 minute to melt the cheeses together.

Add beaten eggs to almond flour, mix well. Combine with the cheese mixture and work until a dough is formed.

Press dough into greased cast iron skillet.
Bake for 10 minutes.

Making the pizza:
Crack eggs onto the dough, and top with all meats and cheeses.
Return to the oven to bake for an additional 10-15 minutes or until set up and golden.

Pesto chicken bakes

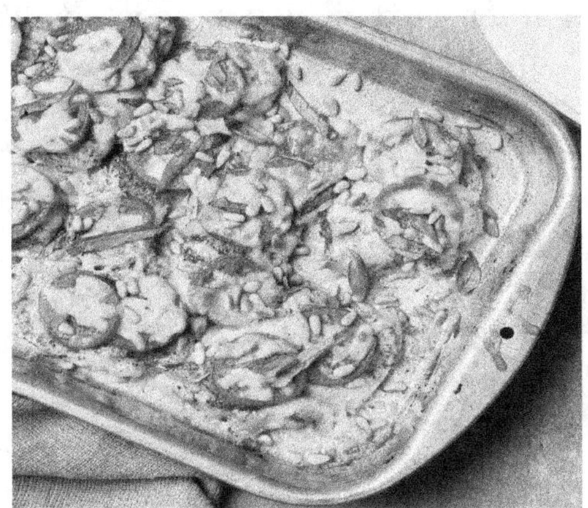

INGREDIENTS

8 (4 ounce) chicken cutlets

½ teaspoon salt

½ teaspoon ground pepper

¼ cup refrigerated basil pesto (such as Buitoni)

4 medium plum tomatoes, sliced

1 ½ cups shredded whole-milk mozzarella cheese

¼ cup thinly sliced fresh basil

2 tablespoons pine nuts, lightly toasted

Place rack in top third of oven; preheat to 425 degrees F. Coat a large rimmed baking sheet with cooking spray. Arrange chicken in a single layer on the baking sheet. Sprinkle the chicken with salt and pepper and spread evenly with pesto. Top with tomato slices and cheese.

Bake until the chicken is cooked through and the cheese is lightly browned and bubbly, 18 to 20 minutes. Top with basil and pine nuts. Serve immediately.

Cheesesteak Roll up

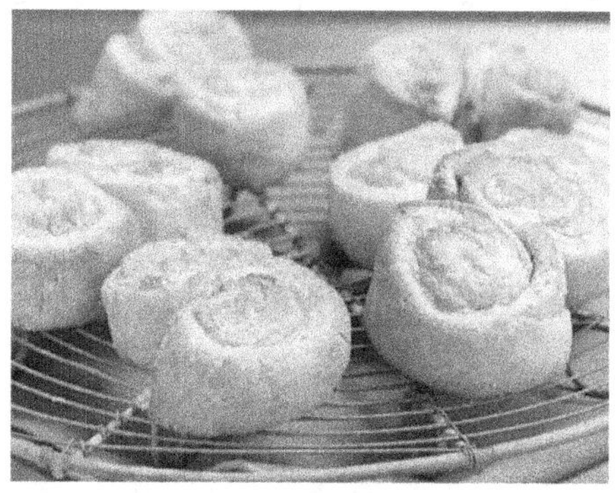

INGREDIENTS

200g self-raising flour, plus extra for dusting
50g butter, softened
1 tsp paprika
100-125ml/3½-4fl oz milk
50g ready-grated mature cheddar

INSTRUCTIONS

Heat oven to 220C/200C fan/gas 7. Put the flour and butter in a bowl and rub them together with your fingers. Rubbing in mixture with cold butter is hard and tiring on young fingers, so use slightly softened butter – but not so soft that it is oily. Now stir in the paprika and mix again.

Add 100ml milk and mix with a fork until you get a soft dough. Add a splash more milk if the dough is dry. This process will teach you how to feel the dough and decide if it needs more liquid. You can always add more milk if required.

On a lightly floured surface, roll out the dough like pastry to about 0.5cm thick. Try to keep a rectangular shape. Only roll in one direction, and roll and turn, roll and turn by keeping the dough moving, you avoid finding it stuck at the end.

Sprinkle the grated cheese on top, then roll up like a sausage along the long side. Cut into 12 thick rings using a table knife. Get an adult to show you how to hold the dough with one hand and cut straight through with the other.

Line the baking tray with baking parchment. Place the roll-ups on the parchment, cut-side down, almost touching each other, making sure that you can see the spiral. Get an adult to put them in the oven for you and bake for 20-25 mins until golden and melty. Ask an adult to remove them from the oven, then leave to cool. The cheese roll-ups will keep for up to 3 days in an airtight container.

CHAPTER: 8 Dinner ideals
Keto bread

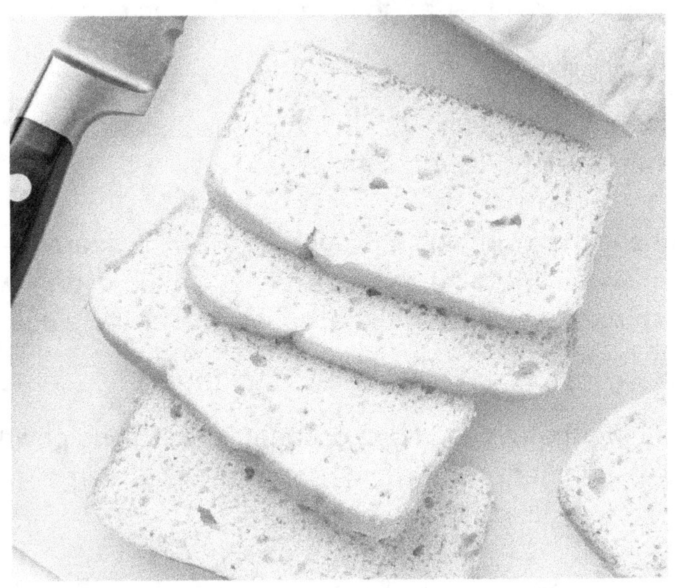

INGREDIENTS
BASIC INGREDIENTS
1 cup Wholesome Yum Blanched Almond Flour
1/4 cup Wholesome Yum Coconut Flour
2 tsp Baking powder
1/4 tsp Sea salt
1/3 cup Unsalted butter (or 5 tbsp + 1 tsp; measured solid, then melted; can use coconut oil for dairy-free)
12 large Egg whites (~1 1/2 cups, at room temperature)

OPTIONAL INGREDIENTS (RECOMMENDED)

1 tbsp Besti Monk Fruit Allulose Blend (can use any sweetener or omit)
1/4 tsp Xanthan gum (for texture – omit for paleo)
1/4 tsp Cream of tartar (to more easily whip egg whites)

INSTRUCTIONS

Tap on the times in the instructions below to start a kitchen timer while you cook.

Preheat the oven to 325 degrees F (163 degrees C). Line an 8 1/2 x 4 1/2 in (22×11 cm) loaf pan with parchment paper, with extra hanging over the sides for easy removal later.

Combine the almond flour, coconut flour, baking powder, Besti, xanthan gum, and sea salt in a large food processor. Pulse until combined.

Add the melted butter. Pulse, scraping down the sides as needed, until crumbly.

In a very large bowl, use a hand mixer to beat the egg whites and cream of tartar (if using), until stiff peaks form. Make sure the bowl is large enough because the whites will expand a lot.

Add 1/2 of the stiff egg whites to the food processor. Pulse a few times until just combined. Do not over-mix!

Carefully transfer the mixture from the food processor into the bowl with the egg whites, and gently fold until no streaks remain. Do not stir. Fold gently to keep the mixture as fluffy as possible.

Transfer the batter to the lined loaf pan and smooth the top. Push the batter toward the center a bit to round the top.

Bake for about 40 minutes, until the top is golden brown. Tent the top with aluminum foil and bake for another 30-45 minutes, until the top is firm and does not make a squishy sound when pressed. Internal temperature should be 200 degrees. Cool completely before removing from the pan and slicing.

Keto fish and chip

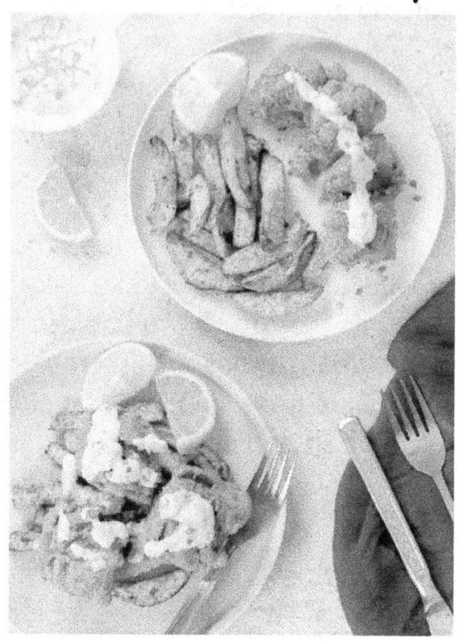

INGREDIENTS
CHIPS
1 medium-large celeriac
2 tablespoon olive oil
¼ teaspoon sage powder
¼ teaspoon cayenne
¼ teaspoon garlic powder
¼ teaspoon onion powder
Salt
Pepper
FISH
½ cup almond flour

1 medium egg
4 tablespoon sparkling water
12 oz / (340 g) whiting fish fillet, cut into big chunks
¼ teaspoon sage powder
¼ teaspoon cayenne
Salt
Pepper
Vegetable oil for frying

INSTRUCTIONS

Put the celeriac sticks in a baking tray lined with waxed paper. Remove excess water from the celeriac with a paper towel.

Sprinkle salt, pepper, cayenne, sage powder, onion powder, and garlic powder on the celeriac. Drizzle with olive oil. Mix gently with your hands until well coated.

Bake the celeriac in a preheated oven at 200°C/390°F fan, for about 25-30 minutes.

Whisk the egg, sparkling water, and almond flour in a large mixing bowl. Set aside.

Heat the vegetable oil in a cast-iron pot for deep frying.

Meanwhile, season the fish filets with salt, pepper, sage powder, and cayenne.

Dip the seasoned fish filets into the almond flour batter, and cover all sides.

Deep fry the fish pieces until slightly golden brown and crisp on each side.

Serve fish and celeriac chips warm with your favorite tartar sauce.

Thai red curry beef with broccoli rice

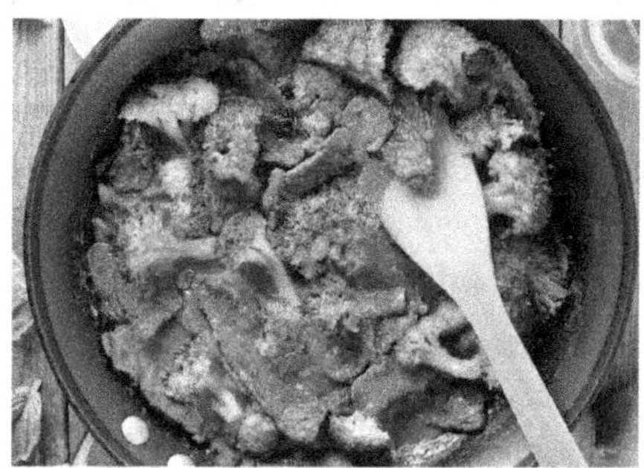

INGREDIENTS

12 ounces broccoli florets (1 1/2 inch florets) - one medium sized head of broccoli

1 tablespoon safflower oil, or olive oil

1 pound beef tenderloin trimmed of any fat (about 2 small filet steaks)

1/2 teaspoon salt & pepper

2 large shallots, thinly sliced

3 tablespoons minced fresh ginger (or substitute with 3/4 teaspoon ground ginger)

1 1/2 tablespoons Thai red curry paste
14 ounces lite coconut milk, stirred thoroughly (one 13.5-oz can)
1 tablespoon firmly packed brown sugar
1 tablespoon Asian fish sauce
steamed Jasmine rice, for serving
8 fresh basil leaves, chopped or torn
4 lime wedges, for serving

INSTRUCTIONS

Steam broccoli on stove-top for approx 13-15 minutes. Avoid overcooking!

While steaming broccoli, slice the shallots, and prepare the beef.

Slice the filet against the grain, very thinly, to create delicate strips about 1/4 inch thick. Lay them flat on a cutting board, cover with plastic wrap, and gently flatten them with a meat tenderizer. (Be very careful when flattening the meat; I literally only pound each section of each piece one time. This ensures a wonderfully tender experience in every bite.) Season the beef slices with salt and pepper.

Sauté the beef in oil in a large sauce pan for about 45 seconds per side. Then transfer to a plate while you continue to cook the rest of the beef in batches. Next add in shallots, sauté for 2-3 minutes, then add ginger for another minute.

Stir in red curry paste and continue to cook for about one more minute. Add in fish sauce, brown sugar, 1/4 teaspoon salt and pepper, and coconut milk, and let it simmer until it thickens up - about 4-5 minutes.
Add your beef and broccoli back into the pan to heat up and serve!

Salmon in Garlic butter with roasted asparagus

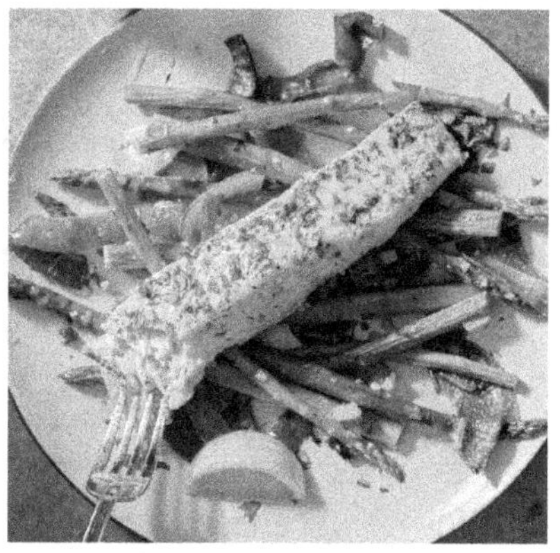

INGREDIENTS
450 g asparagus, trimmed
1 medium red onion, halved, sliced lengthwise into thick wedges
2 tbsp. extra-virgin olive oil
Flaky sea salt
4 salmon filets, skin-on if desired

Freshly ground black pepper

115 g unsalted butter, melted

4 large cloves garlic, finely chopped

2 tbsp. chopped fresh parsley leaves, plus more for serving

3 medium lemons, 1 zested and juiced, 1 juiced, 1 cut into wedges

INSTRUCTIONS

Step 1

Place a rack in top third of oven; preheat to 200°C (180°C Fan). Arrange asparagus on one side of a large rimmed baking tray and onion wedges on the other. Drizzle vegetables with oil; season with salt and toss to coat. Spread vegetables in an even layer, keeping each on their own side of baking tray. Roast until just softened, about 10 minutes.

Step 2

Meanwhile, season salmon with 1 teaspoon salt and 1/4 teaspoon pepper. In a small bowl, mix butter, garlic, parsley, lemon zest, and 3 tablespoons lemon juice; season with salt and pepper.

Step 3

Remove baking tray from oven; push onion to one side and asparagus to the other. Arrange salmon skin side down in centre of baking tray. Spoon about three-quarters of butter mixture over salmon. Spoon remaining butter over vegetables.

Step 4

Bake salmon 8 minutes. Turn on grill and grill on high, watching closely, until salmon is just cooked through and vegetables are tender and browned in spots, 3 to 5 minutes more.

Step 5

Top with parsley. Serve with lemon wedges alongside.

Peanut butter chicken curry

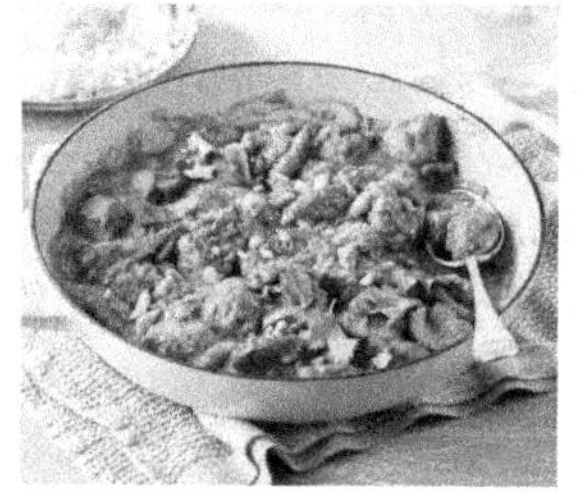

INGREDIENTS

1 large chicken, jointed, or 1.5kg bone-in chicken pieces
6 garlic cloves, 2 finely chopped, 4 left whole
3 lemongrass stalks, bashed and roughly chopped
thumb-sized piece of ginger, peeled and finely chopped
1 tbsp ground cumin
1 tbsp ground coriander
1 tbsp ground turmeric
2 limes, juiced
2 red chillies, 1 roughly chopped and 1 sliced to serve (optional)
1 small onion, roughly chopped

2 tbsp vegetable oil

100g smooth peanut butter

4 tbsp kecap manis, or 3 tbsp soy sauce mixed with 1 tbsp light brown soft sugar

400g can coconut milk

To serve

a few spring onions, chopped

small handful of coriander, chopped

small handful of roasted peanuts, roughly chopped (optional)

INSTRUCTIONS

STEP 1

Put the chicken, chopped garlic, a third of the lemongrass and half the ginger, spices and lime juice in a large bowl. Toss, then cover and leave for 30 mins, or chill for up to 24 hrs. Blitz the whole garlic, the rest of the lemongrass and ginger, remaining spices, chopped chili, onion and a large splash of water to in a food processor. Set aside.

STEP 2

Heat the oil in a pan and brown the chicken all over. Set aside on a plate. Cook the paste for 8-10 mins until it splits. Stir in the peanut butter and kecap manis. When thickened, add the coconut milk and half a can of water, bring to a simmer, season, then add the chicken with its juices. Continue to simmer for 40 mins, stirring often. Turn off the heat, add the rest of the lime juice and season. Leave to rest for 10 mins. Scatter over the sliced chili, spring onions, fresh coriander and peanuts to serve.

Keto pizza

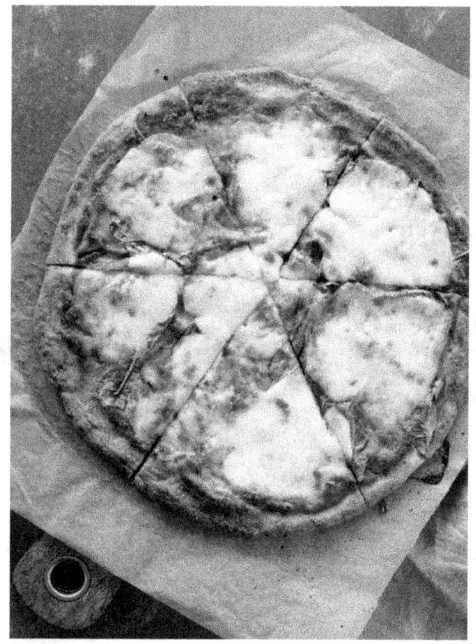

INGREDIENTS
2 cups Shredded Mozzarella Cheese
1 oz cream cheese, (or 2 tablespoons)
1 cup Almond Flour
1 egg
1 teaspoon baking powder
1 teaspoon Italian seasoning, optional
1 teaspoon garlic powder, optional

TOPPINGS

Cheese, shredded mozzarella, fresh mozzarella, parmesan, feta etc
Your favorite meats, chicken, beef, pepperoni, turkey, etc
Your favorite veggies, Onion, Pepper, Jalapeno, olives, spinach, etc
Your favorite sauce, sugar-free tomato sauce, olive oil, ranch, blue cheese, buffalo, etc
Herbs, Parmesan, Crushed Red Peppers
Directions

INSTRUCTIONS

Preheat oven to 450 F.
Add mozzarella and cream cheese to a large microwave-safe bowl and microwave for 45 seconds.

Remove from microwave and add in egg, almond flour, baking powder, Italian seasoning, and garlic. Mix with a spoon until well incorporated.

Transfer dough onto a large piece of parchment paper and cover with another piece of parchment paper. Flatten out dough using a rolling pin to about ¼" thick.

Remove parchment paper and shape with hands if desired.

Transfer pizza on the parchment paper onto a baking sheet or pizza stone and bake for 10 minutes.

Remove from oven (keep the oven on) and load your pizza however you like with all of your favorite sauces, cheese, and toppings.

Bake pizza for another 5-8 minutes or until the cheese is bubbly.

Skirt Steak and Mustard sauce

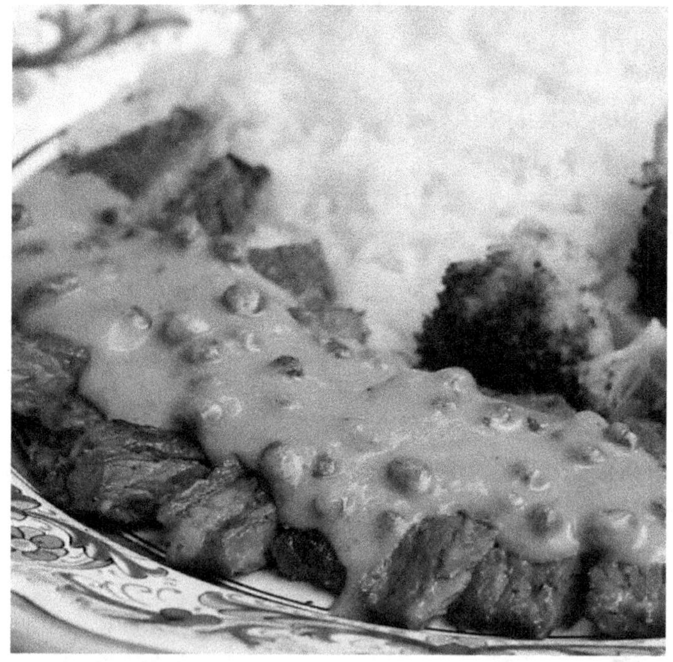

INGREDIENTS
FOR 2 SERVINGS
1 lb skirt steak(455 g), room temperature
1 teaspoon kosher salt

1 teaspoon black pepper
1 ½ tablespoons olive oil
¼ cup beef broth(60 mL)
2 tablespoons dijon mustard
1 tablespoon unsalted butter
1 ½ tablespoons capers in brine
rice, cooked, for serving
broccoli, steamed, for serving

INSTRUCTIONS

Cut steak in half crosswise. Season with the salt and pepper.

Heat the olive oil in a nonstick or stainless steel pan over medium heat for 1 minute. Add 1 portion of steak and cook until a golden brown crust has formed, 4-5 minutes per side. Transfer the seared steak to a plate and repeat with the remaining portion of steak. If the pan is getting too dry, add a bit more olive oil. Let the steaks rest for 3 minutes.

After the steak has rested, transfer to a cutting board and pour any accumulated meat juices from the plate back into the pan and return to medium heat.
Add the beef broth and scrape up any brown bits from the bottom of the pan. Add the mustard and butter and stir until combined. Stir in the capers and cook until the sauce thickens slightly, 1-2 minutes.

Slice the steak into ¼-inch (6 mm) pieces and transfer to serving plates. Pour the sauce over the steak and serve with rice and broccoli.

Enjoy!

CONCLUSION

As you close the last part of "Excursion to the Whole Body Reset recollect that this isn't simply a book; It's your ticket to a fresh start. You've left on a groundbreaking campaign, revealing the key to opening your body's maximum capacity. You've navigated the uncharted waters of self-discovery, mindful nutrition, and energizing exercise, like an expert navigator.

As the book tenderly says goodbye, imagine yourself remaining at the highest point of your own comprehensive victory. The excursion isn't just about resetting your body; it's tied in with reworking your account. You are the creator of a freshly discovered imperativeness, etched by decisions, versatility, and the significant comprehension that genuine wellbeing is a craftsmanship, not an objective.

Embrace the reverberations of strengthening that resound from the pages you've turned. This isn't the end; it's a preamble to a daily existence set apart by recharged energy, balance, and a significant association with the surprising vessel that is your body. The end words might leave the book, however the groundbreaking reverberations of your process will keep on resonating, forming an account of health, versatility, and the victory of taking care of oneself. In this way, as you turn the last page, step into the future - a material anticipating the brushstrokes of your proceeded with Entire Body Reset

ABOUT the AUTHOR

Dr. Sharon S. Lent

Welcome to the realm of sustainable weight loss and nourishing diets! **Dr. Lent,** a seasoned medical professional specializing in weight loss and diet, brings a wealth of expertise to guide you on your transformative journey to a healthier you.

Meet Dr. Sharon S. Lent

With a passion for empowering individuals to achieve their health goals, **Dr. Sharon S. Lent** has dedicated her career to the intersection of medicine, nutrition, and well-being. Holding a Doctor of Medicine degree, her specialized focus on weight loss has allowed her to make a meaningful impact on countless lives.

Areas of Expertise

Dr. Lent is renowned for her comprehensive approach to weight management, combining medical knowledge with practical, sustainable strategies. Her expertise includes personalized diet plans, evidence-based interventions, and holistic well-being practices.

A Trusted Guide:

As a trusted guide on the journey to better health, **Dr. Lent** emphasizes the importance of mindful living, making choices that resonate with individual lifestyles, and fostering a positive relationship with food.

Contributions to the Field:

Beyond her clinical practice, **Dr. Lent** is an avid contributor to the field of weight management. Her research, articles, and contributions to reputable health publications reflect a commitment to sharing knowledge and fostering a community dedicated to wellness.

Join the Journey:

Embark on a journey towards sustainable weight loss and a nourished, balanced life with **Dr. Lent**. Through her insights, you'll discover practical, achievable steps that go beyond the conventional approach to dieting, paving the way for a healthier, more vibrant future.

Review

Dear **Reader,**

We hope you're enjoying your journey with the **"Total Health Transformation"** Your experience matters to us, and we'd love to hear your thoughts on how the program has been for you.

Whether you've just started or are well into your transformation, your review can inspire others and help us fine-tune our approach to better suit your needs. Please take a moment to share your feedback on the **"Total Health Transformation"**. Your insights are invaluable in shaping the success stories of our community.

Thank you for being a part of this journey with us. Your review is not just a reflection of your experience but also a beacon for others seeking a healthier lifestyle.

We appreciate your time and input.